WHY DO WE CONDUCT RESEARCH THE WAY WE DO?

Research in nursing, a logical-philosophical reflection

Marcos Renato de Oliveira, RN, Ph.D.

CONTENT

ABSTRACT

This book presents a critical reflection on nursing research practices, from a logical-philosophical perspective. The competence of a researcher requires development of scientific spirit and the follow-up of the precepts of logic. The present material is based on the critical reflection method. The findings of this book allows us to review our own research practices and to identify that despite the fact that science is dynamic, the practice of research conducting is not so dynamic. Furthermore, in order to pursue the practice of nursing it is necessary to be aware of the principles and basis of scientific practice. I hope to contribute to the stimulus to critical (re)thinking about nursing research practices and their continuation presented here can provide the advancement of nursing as a science which will consequently provide social improvements instead of reproduction of methods and personal satisfaction.

Keywords: Nursing research, Logic, Philosophy of Science.

INTRODUCTION

Many nurses have been providing not just clinical care; many also become scientists who are looking for a better practice. However, are nursing scientists just following methods or are we really promoting improvement for society? Also, why do we conduct research, and the respective analyses of data in the way we do?

For a proper understanding of nursing research practice a discussion about the logic applied to the research method is pertinent. In view of this, this book presents a critical reflection that aims to discuss nursing research practices.

In regard to truth and its concept throughout history, we emphasize that among the most accepted theories today, truth is actually grouped into what is said, what is felt, what is intuited and what is informed by our senses. The first two, especially the truth that we are told, allude directly to authority, formerly closely linked to religious and political truths, are nowadays very present in the academic world. However, the truth of senses, to be mediated by the perception, selectivity and capacity of interpretation, among the observation of other precepts, is an important key for the practice of research and experimentation. This is due to that fact the scientific truth understood as a reality is constructed by observing the precepts of science and by the use of theories and instruments simultaneously[1].

Moreover, it is well known that the science of logic was first described by the Greeks. Aristotle had molded this study in the form of syllogism, whose exactness of the syllogistic process is fixed in eight fundamental rules. The proper follow-up of these premises will allow researchers to deduce a conclusion and to develop a perfect logical argument.

While observing the first studies of the sciences, we can perceive that they look for the identification, observation, analysis, and reproduction of events, at least to understand the law that governs events. However, analyzing the above information leads us to understand that the problem of knowledge is a complex problem whose main aspects refer to the structuring, value, and correct functioning of scientific research practices. Therefore, although the reflexive process had been increasingly valued, there are few publications that explain how to use it in favor of promoting a development in health education. It is necessary to understand that health practice is interdisciplinary, which gives it an integrative characteristic of knowledge and skills, coupled with ethical and political attitudes so necessary to professional competence in nursing[2].

Today it is easy to see that the main problems in nursing researchers include weak or poorly implemented designs and predictable or well-known findings. Some had a combination of these. Weak designs included use of untested measures, inadequate samples, descriptive or cross-sectional designs in support of claims of prediction or causality, and weak or incomplete qualitative analyses[3].

It is up to researchers, from the very beginning of nursing as a science, to strengthen the practices by the intellect, due to the fact that nursing practice descends from human knowledge and that it is necessary to mention that human knowledge has basic differences that make it completely different from that of other species, such as the presence of memory and fantasy. Therefore, the present book aims to perform a critical reflection on nursing research practices, from a logical-philosophical perspective. I hope to stimulate nursing researchers to discuss their own research practices and the need to conduct research practices based on the principles of science.

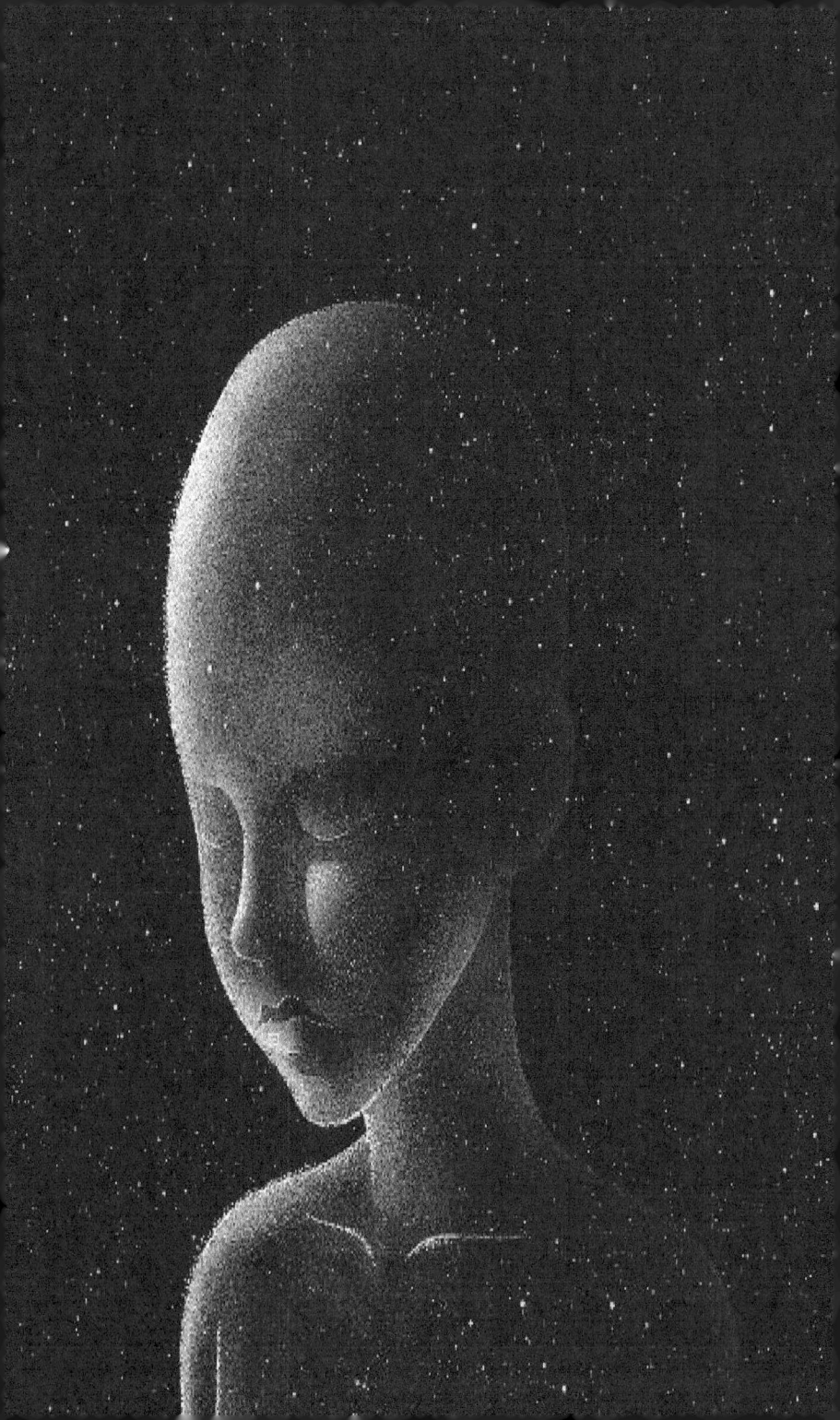

METHODS

The present book is based on the critical reflection method. This type of reflection aims to renew the ways of thinking about and executing health practices, with the ultimate goal of intervention in social reality in order to improve the living and health conditions of communities[2].

For a critical understanding, I agree with Duncan (2007) that in order to develop a critical analysis, this analysis must occur outside of the system, while many of the fatuous practices may be the fruits of the very system in which we are subjected[4]. Thus, I have not demeaned my previous methods and publications but I have reflected on my own research practices, based on philosophical texts, and I have adopted the understanding of science as the area of knowledge of things by causes[5].

RESULTS AND DISCUSSION

When analyzing nursing research I was faced with the fact that the practice of research is an older act than the execution of the nursing practice itself as a formal profession. I could also identify that: in order to be scientists we need to use many principles of philosophy, especially the fundamentals of the principles of logic. Thus, in order to facilitate the presentation of results and discussion, I present my results in detailed topics: the logical problem and the gnosiological problem (knowledge problem), Aristotle and the first Western systematization of knowledge, the origin of current practices of care and research, and Popper's contribution to nursing practices in research.

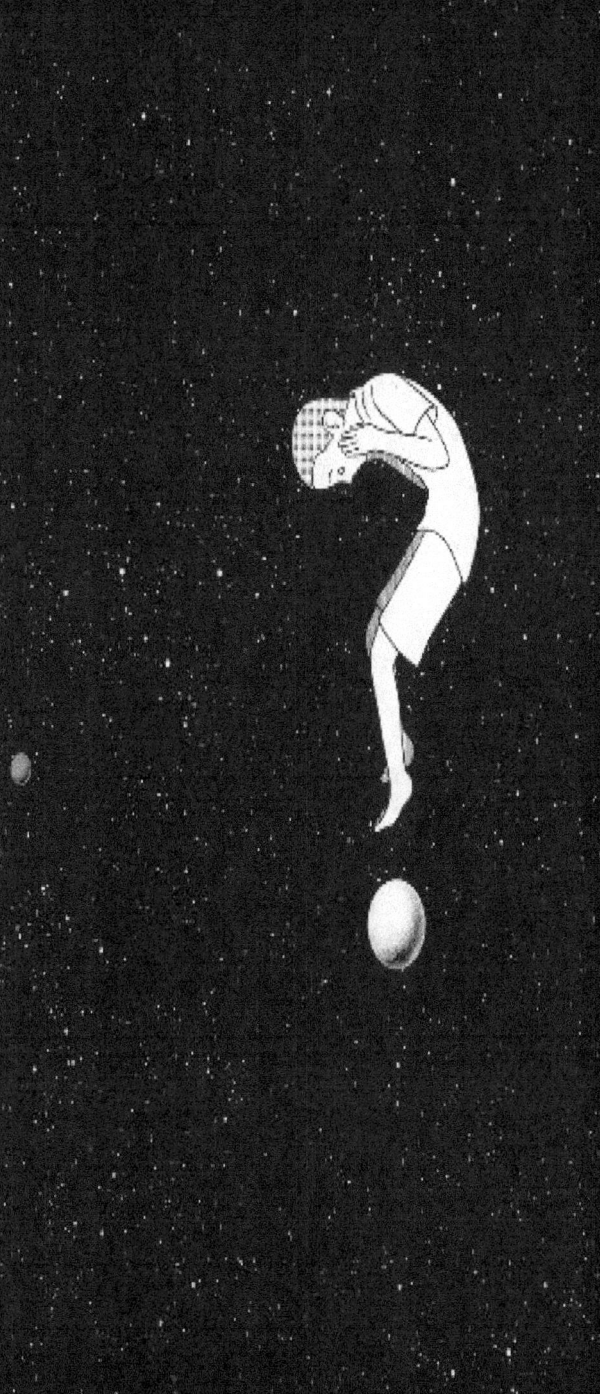

The logical problem and the gnosiological problem (knowledge problem)

Human knowledge is an area of interest in gnosiology and logic. Of these, logic stands out, understood as the science that studies thought while thinking, while attaching attention to the object and not to the representation of the idea. This science is divided into three main branches: formal logic, transcendental logic and mathematical logic.

The thinker Kant elaborated on transcendental logic, in which the elements that constitute the truth of science were investigated. This was acclaimed by many while it was also criticized and rejected by several other researchers.

Regarding the origin of ideas, it is known that there are two forms of knowledge, the sensitive and the intellective, where it can be inferred that all knowledge is produced by the object and the subject. It is also possible to say that intellect is produced by the subject and sensible by the object. Therefore, the intellectual knowledge is the result of the joint action of the subject and the object. Furthermore, it is argued that intellective knowledge is produced by the object and sensible by the subject and that sensible knowledge and intellectual knowledge are both the result of the ideal joint action of the subject and the object, according to Plato, Hegel, Occam, Berkeley, Aristotle and Kant.

At first, it is necessary to emphasize that the nurse who proposes to be a researcher/scientist, besides having a solid moral formation, must have a series of qualities that are not found in common subjects such as independence of thought, positive spirit, impartiality, disinterested thinking, faith in science, and a sense of social responsibility[5].

According to Descartes, it is not enough to have a scientific profile if one does not know how to apply well the knowledge that one has. Thus, the use of the scientific method proposed by Descartes, which consists of four macro rules, is made pertinent: to admit only what becomes intrinsically evident; to divide the difficulties in order to better solve them; to order the thoughts, beginning with the simplest ones to rise gradually, to the more complex ones; and, last but not least, and to enumerate all the phenomena approached, so that all objects/subjects are properly studied and understood in their essence and not in the scientist's view[5].

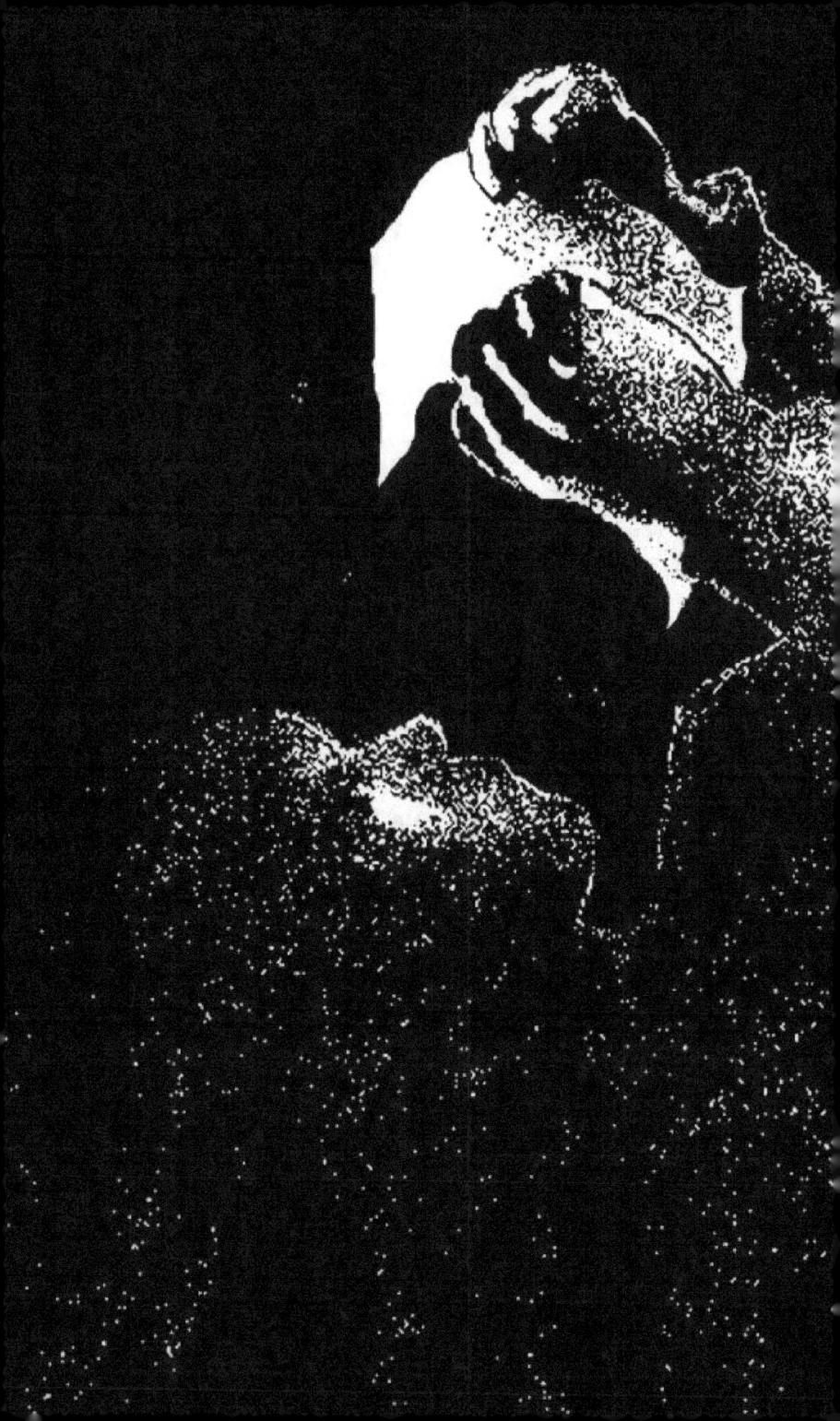

Aristotle and the first Western systematization of knowledge

Aristotle was born in 384/383 BC, by the Macedonian border. He was the son of a physician and at the age of 18 entered the Platonic academy, where he assimilated his principles and moved to new heights. He left the academy due to private beliefs and in 343/342 BC, taught Alexander the son of Philip of Macedon from Greece, and died in 322 BC. C., after only a few months of exile[6]. His writings are divided into two large groups, the exoteric and the esoteric, and his most famous work consists of fourteen books of metaphysics. Between Plato and Aristotle there are basically two great differences: in Aristotle's interests, Aristotle was interested in almost all empirical sciences, while Plato had an interest in mathematical sciences, and the second difference lies in the fact that Aristotle was systematic in his ideas, while Plato was ironic.

Metaphysics was presented by Aristotle as the search of the first causes and concerns supersensible substance. Aristotle said that the principle must be eternal and in as much as the movement is eternal, everlasting should be the cause. The Principle must be immovable; in fact, only the property is absolute cause of the action, where everything that is in movement is moved by another. Thirdly, this Principle must be entirely deprived of potentiality, that is, pure act. From this he concluded that the world had no beginning, there was not a moment when there was chaos, precisely because, if there were, it would contradict the theorem of the priority of the act over power.

However, Aristotle did not intend to deny the existence of supra-sensible realities but simply to deny that the supra-sensible was what Plato thought it to be. Whereas the world of the supersensible is not the world of the intelligible, but of intelligences, being in its vertex the supreme of the intelligences, due to the fact that ideas or forms, are verified by the intelligible plot of the sensible.

The influence of Aristotle for the practice of research is enormous, even having deepened still further the question of movement, establishing the forms of the movement and the ontological structure, also he discussed about time and denied that there was an infinite in an act.

It is also known that Aristotelian´s physics does not investigate only the physical universe but also the beings that are in the universe, especially the animate beings, humans. By that the fundamental phenomena and functions of life are the vegetative character, the sensory-motor character, and the intellectual character. Thus, for these reasons, Aristotle introduced the distinction between the vegetative soul, the sensitive soul, and the intellective or rational soul[1].

Next to the theoretical sciences come the practical sciences. The study of conduct or the end of man as an individual is ethics; the study of conduct and the end of man as part of a society is politics. Both lead man to his supreme end, happiness[1].

In this context, logic arises to show how thought proceeds when thinking, what is the structure are elements of reasoning, how to present demonstrations, what are the types and modes of demonstration, what and when something can be demonstrated[5].

Generally, in perfect reasoning there must be three propositions, of which two of those functions are antecedents, so they are called premises, and the third is consequent of what arises in this premises. There is a classic example of the syllogism: if all men are mortal, and if Socrates is man, then Socrates is mortal[5].

Aristotle says that induction and intuition are processes in a sense opposed to the syllogistic process but are presupposed by the syllogism in itself. In face of these facts, we also emphasize that it is still necessary for the researchers to clearly understand what is scientific and what is just a technical activity. Despite the confusion among the general public, the concepts are different.

Science is placed at the disposal of the society while technology is at the disposal of our needs. Science seeks to know things for what they are and technology seeks to produce what we want it to be[1]. When we think of research, besides following a method and appropriate instruments, we must use common sense, understood as a kind of innate logic which is found at different levels of development in all individuals[5].

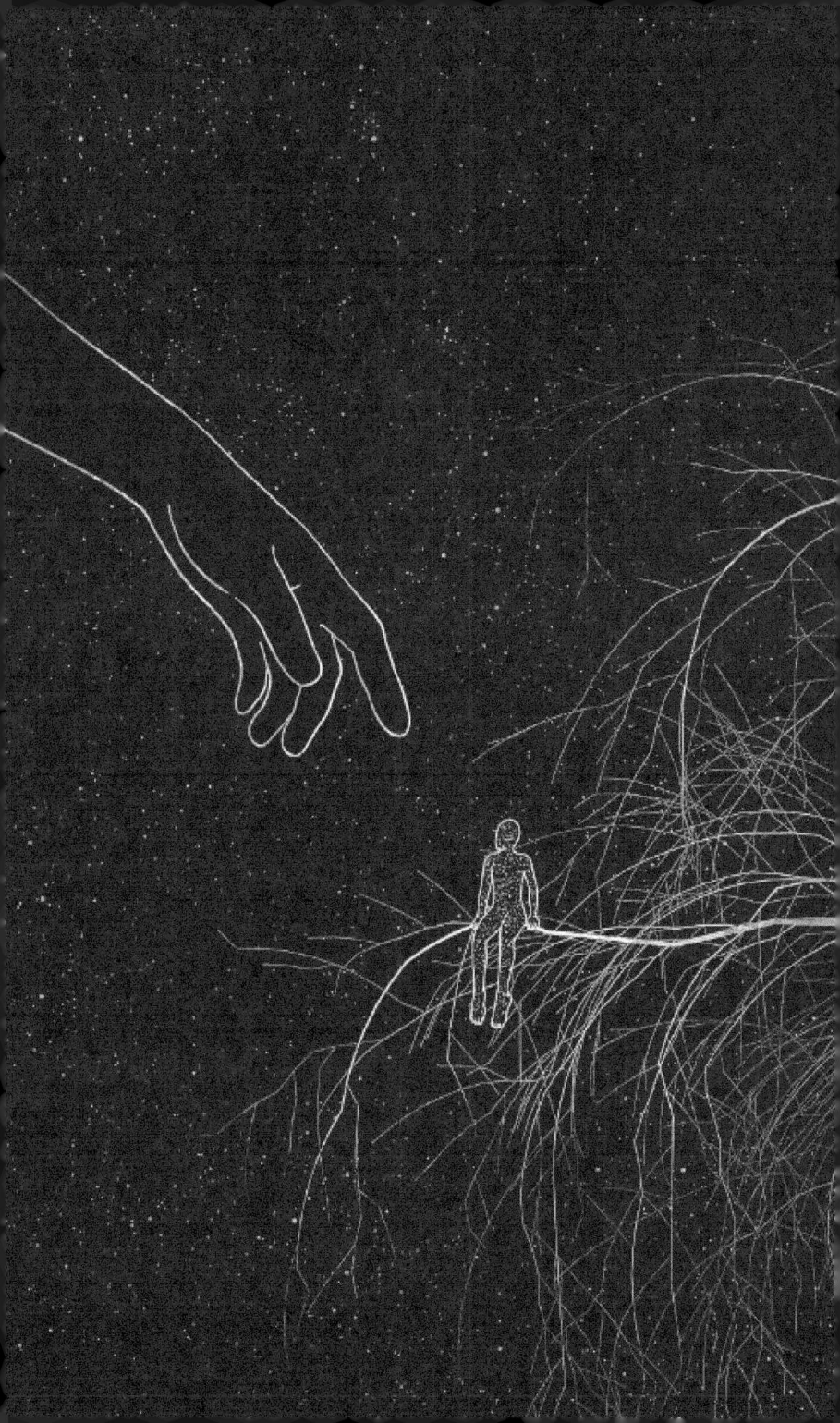

The origin of current practices
of care and investigation

The Renaissance was a period marked by the blooming and spread of various ideals and ideas but it can be said that it was a time less endowed with a critical spirit. It was a period wrapped in superstition, a fact proved by the analysis of the literature of that period and the lack of critical spirit resulting from the destruction of the Aristotelian ontology[7].

Associated with this set of factors, the fact that stands out is that human is a credulous animal by nature, believing in stories passed on and in facts seen, we emphasize that the great majority are not perceived, only seen. So while the human does not perceive magic as absurd, there is only reason to believe this practice, and if observed closely, always in every belief, deep down there is a magic ontology. What sums up the Renaissance in a single sentence: anything is possible.

However, the other side of the same period, that of curiosity, which allowed the exploration of lands beyond previously unexplored horizons, categorization of new species, study of the human body, and mathematics itself, is undeniable. It should also be noted that many of these studies only occurred as categorization rather than classification. Furthermore, it was Roger Bacon who was responsible for putting experimental science on a very high plane, studying and multiplying the ideas of deductive reasoning, leading to the conclusion that the only criterion of truth would be logical coherence, and experimental verification. The question of why things occurred in this period have been replaced by how things happened. However, it should be noted that the great revolution of this period was due to scientific thought, not to the evolution of inventions, as these were fruits of practical necessity.

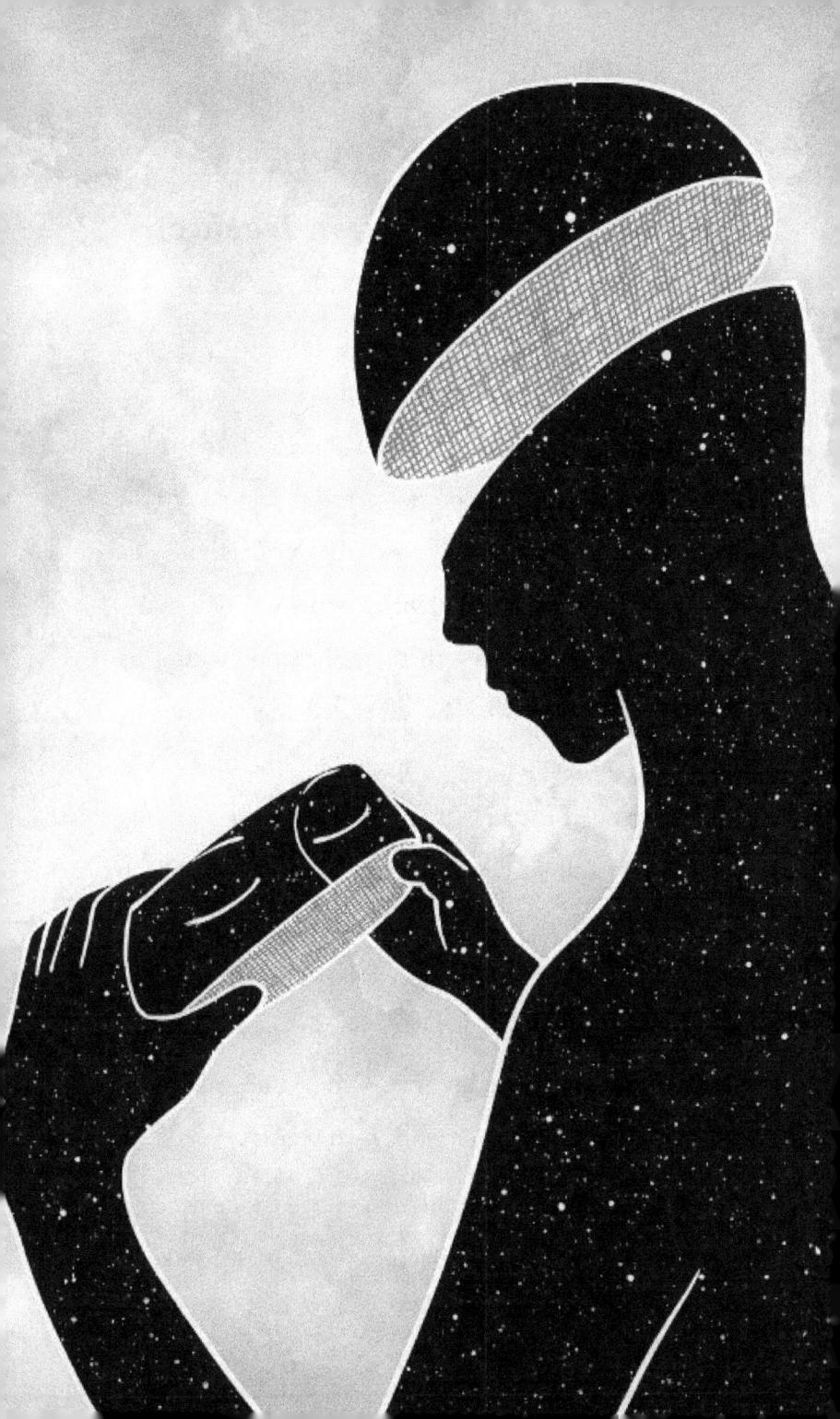

Popper's contribution to nursing practices in research

Although philosophical literature brings the image of Popper associated with neopositivism, in our conception, we do not perceive it as positivist, while replacing the principle of verification with the principle of falsifiability. Popper was one of the most courageous theoretical opponents of totalitarianism who he defended metaphysics as the progenitor of scientific theories and maintained the idea that the best theories are the least probable. This gave him the reputation of the official opposition of the Vienna Circle. The idea that humans should stop worrying about words and their meanings in order to start worrying about theories of criticism, reasoning, and validity is pointed out in the author's own words[8].

The assertion that induction does not exist, and that the opposite conception is a big mistake is

Popper's answer to the problem of induction. As such, it states that it is of a repetitive nature or of elimination. The idea of induction must be eliminated because there are no methods based on routine or nothing that can be affirmed simply by denying contrary statements[6].

Still, Popper states that from the logical point of view it is not at all obvious that it is justified to infer universal assertions from singular assertions, however numerous the latter. In such a way that any conclusion drawn in this way can always prove to be false, an example is known to us: however, many white swans we may have observed, does not justify the conclusion that all swans are white[8].

Starting from the particular case of nursing practice, it is common to use data inference and particular cases for the universal population; we believe that some authors do this in an innocent way, by not observing the aforementioned principles, or perhaps by a limited and immature view of the universe and its aspects. On the other hand, other researchers make inferences under the shield of mathematics where it attempts to prove that what is found is a mirror of what happens in other populations with similar characteristics including justifications that seem logical for most of the public. Often these analyses do not follow the principles of logic in research. However, it should be pointed out that although the idea that replicating situations under similar conditions generates similar results is false, it can be a false assertion when it is directed towards humans, considering that they are social beings.

For Popper, observtivism is a philosophical myth, for we are not clean slate. Humans are full of signs and marks from cultural evolution. Therefore, an experiment or proof always presupposes a hypothesis that we create in order to solve problems. In this way, Popper destroys the position of all who maintained and maintain that observation must precede expectations and problems[8].

Some philosophical strands claim that we have inductive knowledge and others that we absorb through observation of the world even though we are not empty of concepts and ideas about what we perceive. Further, we can´t empty ourselves of our ideas of the world when we cast our gaze on it, which infers us to say, as well as Popper, that the observtivism is a myth.

Thus, believing that research starts with problems and that to solve them it is necessary to elaborate hypotheses must be proved by the falsification. The detail is in the fact that if it is not possible to extract from a theory of consequences that can be verified as factual, they are not scientific. Popper still argued for the idea that a scientific system was not required to be chosen positively once and for all but it was required that its logical form be such that it can be verified through empirical evidence, in the negative sense an empirical system must be able to be refuted by experience[6].

In observing Popper's points, we realized that he believed that it was the goal of science to reach ever more credible theories, always inching closer to the truth. While science seeks truth, so this truth is not given by facts but by theories and that a theory is true when it corresponds to the facts. On the other hand, to say that an assertion or a set of assertions is not scientific does not imply that it is foolish[8].

The first impression seems contradictory, to say that scientific discovery is impossible without faith, what to say then of speculative atomism and of so many other ideas and principles, which are now reproduced experimentally but were born of the observation and ordering of human images. It is a fact that there are sensible theories and these, although they are empirically irrefutable, can be criticized[6].

Already attributed to Albert Einstein, the phrase that nothing is completely explained without faith, not even science, in this text, I as author, do not refer to faith as belief in God or gods but faith as the act of believing in the impalpable and impossible to experience[6]. Thus, as Popper cites about speculative atomism, or even taking as an example the theories of creation of the universe or still, they are those of the end of the universe, the one that we still live, in although they are reproduced, although in part and in proportion almost by insignificant, they survive by the faith that they are real in other proportions and in other times never before experienced by those who have them as truth. What would that be if not faith?

Finally, we observe that Popper is a contemporary philosopher with extremely rich and practical ideas for the organization and better development of a developed society. The researcher needs to start from obvious and certain principles in order to analyze and reduce to the simplest elements every question to be solved. To reach the adequate scientific profile, it is indispensable to eliminate from knowledge the unconscious psychological projections of the researcher himself on the universe[1]. Also, the pleasure that a researcher generates will inevitably come about as a casual consequence of what he/she did, not as effect that the action constitutes[9].

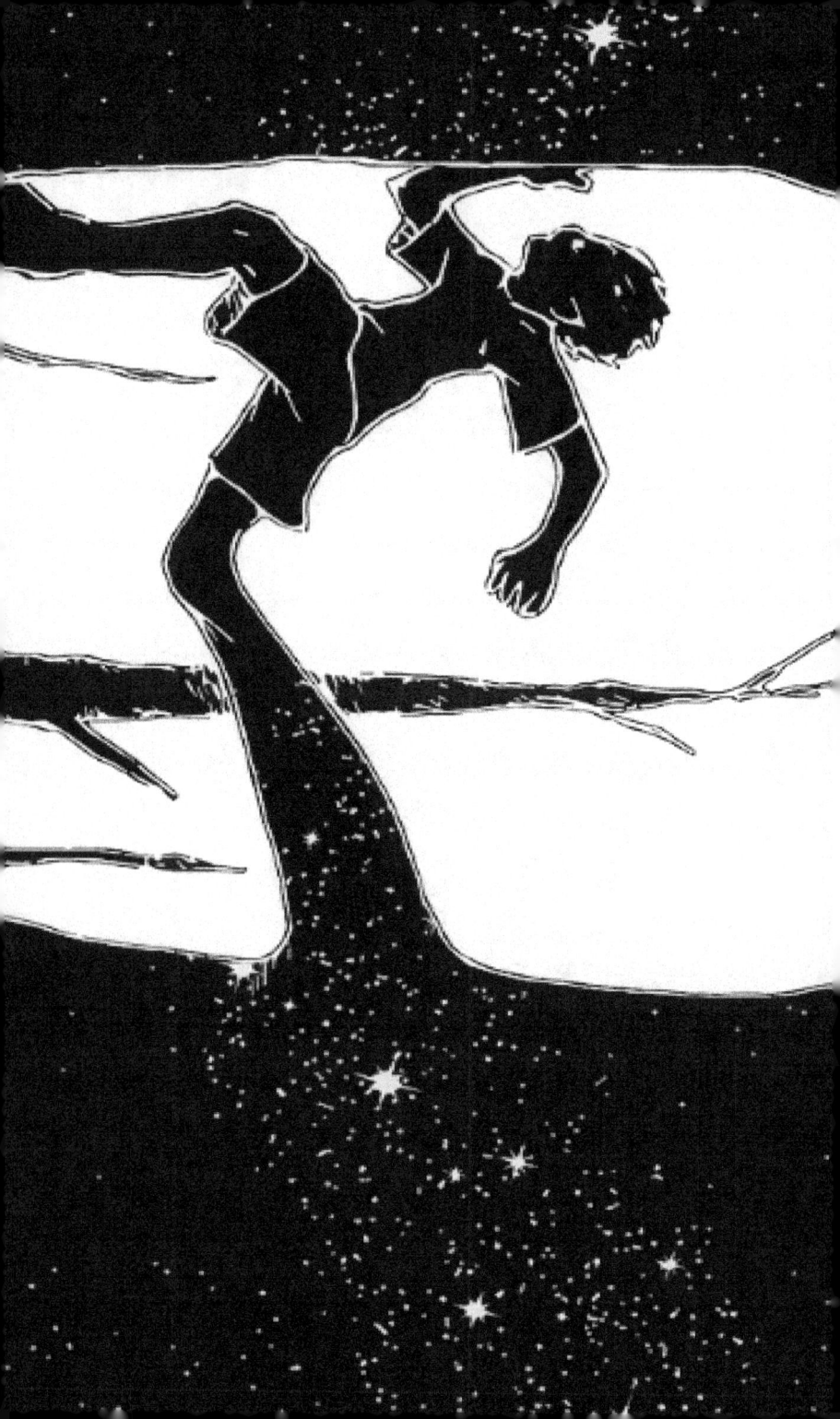

FINAL

CONSIDERATIONS

When reflecting on the practice of nursing research, it is necessary to emphasize something logical, that the same is done by humans. However, much is questioned about the value of human knowledge and effective methods of securing knowledge and obtaining the truth. Both are defended respectively by members of the clergy and by scientists, and obviously, the object of several philosophers throughout history.

It is interesting to note that the research is not part of observations but always of problems, whereas what we, researchers, research precisely the solution to problems and for this, it becomes necessary to use creativity, followed by proof. It is necessary to understand that the falsification of a theory leads to the enrichment of problems. Thus, in the face of all falsified theory, instead of introducing *ad hoc* hypotheses, we must ask: why is this? And finding the answer, this will be precisely a better theory than the falsified theory. For it will be able to explain also those facts or observations that have falsified the previous theory. The epistemology proposes to answer what the scientific knowledge is, in its variables, counting on the help of the neopositivists that divide the sciences in two great branches, the mathematical logic, and the experimental one.

Finally, care must be taken in using our findings. While the historical review of our practices shows us easily how far the conception of reality is ephemeral, and that nothing is static, but dynamic, everything is constantly changing, especially the research practices themselves. It is also necessary that media, academic journals, and regulatory agencies and financiers of the development of science, be sensitive to the practice of science by science and not to the satisfaction of economic and individual interests. We invite nurses, researchers, and other members of society to observe the precepts raised here and reflect on research practices, whether they are science, aimed at social development, or whether they are only a reproduction of methods, aimed at the satisfaction of the personal interest.

REFERENCES

1. Huisman, D., & Vergez, A. (1970). Modern philosophy course: introduction to the philosophy of science. Freitas Bastos.

2. Burgatti, J. C., Leonello, V. M., Bracialli, L. A. D., & Oliveira, M. A. C. (2013). Pedagogical strategies for developing ethical and political competence in nursing education. *Revista Brasileira de Enfermagem, 66*(2), 282-286.

3. Kearney, M. H. (2017). Making Dissertations Publishable. Res Nurs Health, 40: 3–5. doi:10.1002/nur.21780

4. Duncan, P. (2007). Critical perspectives on health. Basingstoke [England]: Palgrave Macmillan.

5. Mortari, C. A. (2001). *Introduction to logic*. SciELO-Editora UNESP.

6. Antiseri, D., & Reale, G. (1990). History of philosophy. *São Paulo: Paulus, 2.*

7. Koiré, A. (1982). History of scientific thought studies. Forense Universitária.

8. Neiva, E. (1999). Popper's criticial rationalism. Francisco Alves.

9. Pettit, P. (2018). Three mistakes about doing good (and bad). *Journal of Applied Philosophy, 35*(1), 1-25.